BROKEN SYNTAX

Laura Hargrove Schneilin

'One million people commit suicide every year.'
The World Health Organization

Published by
Chipmunkapublishing
PO Box 6872
Brentwood
Essex CM13 1ZT
United Kingdom

http://www.chipmunkapublishing.com

BROKEN SYNTAX

To Dr Antoine Jolivet

Laura Hargrove Schneilin

I. Fractures

I. Fractures

Laura Hargrove Schneilin

Redux

I wish I had
Endured
Everything, my life
Strangeness
And death,
Without a blemish.
I wish I stared
Blandness
In the morning
Mirror
Surviving unscathed.
But then my face
Is marked by you,
Brother, lover,
Whoever,
Time, past, friend.
I wish I had
Never been hurt,
Never been
Touched at all.

Laura Hargrove Schneilin

E.D.

The funeral lasted
Through the night
They came and went
For their own delight.

The funeral ended
Without fright
The tears were spent
And then came light.

Grazing

The lonely livestock
Stood part of me
Of my mythology.

Bored of this of lack of pain
My feelings – cattle, swine –
Even so will not subside.

Ode: Wanderlust

The wanderer – my germ,
I named him –
Just for the record had eyes
Like a bowl of risks and teeth
Kept hidden.

The last week I remembered
Cathedrals vanishing
On his forehead
Jutting out
From his hips bones
Building futile castles,
The bruised shadow of his smile
Spreading north south
All over my mind
And the capital.

Syntax

Broken words
Strewn all around
You pick them
Up
And we make Sounds
Broken syntax
Soon heals
Our broken words.

Laura Hargrove Schneilin

A Smile in the Shadow

In the beginning
Came the smile
And the smile and
The Eyes
Were within mine
Then the smile faded
And I was emptied
And ripped apart
And a big gap
Is now my mouth
Still standing
Where the eyes
Used to smile.

Clockwork

If I could think
Louder than the words
That go tick tick
Through the heart
I could find the time
In the body in the bones
To watch an hour
Maybe grow
Grow slowly fearlessly.

Laura Hargrove Schneilin

Disjointed

A mess of words
Four by four
Grapple to find
Meaning in sound.
They are lost now
When
The mind falters
But left to grow
Alone
When thought and sinews
Rejoin and recoup.

God's own Sewing

Is it too late
To mend
A broken heart?
Heart broken
By time too heavy
To bear alone
By moments too clear
To see in the light
And by feelings frozen
In flesh and marrow.

One Day at a Time

Every time
I see
You
I sense
You
Again
Love or hate
You
Again
Last time
First time
Remembered
Too clearly
It's always
You
I can't
Forget.

Paralysis

Sometimes she felt
So cold
And so hungry
And so deserted
That nothing
Could quench
The thirst
That turned
To burning
Inside and out.
And sometimes
She wondered
If the searing
Had any meaning
At all.

Laura Hargrove Schneilin

Mourning

There is the dullness
Of lead
The dullness
Of the foggy Paris winter
No hope
But dread
Of more to come.

There is the dread
Of the dullness
Of the sky now atrophied
And the long long
Sinking
Into bleak winter's despair.

Ghosts

Tomorrow could be blessed
Or meaningless
A frown – a smile –
A figure from behind
Speechless and demure
Looking tiny and forlorn
Brings back the past so fast
Again – It could last or
Disappear, again.

Laura Hargrove Schneilin

Small Victories

On a drab drab winter day
I thought that death
Had come to stay.
So I thought, and sought
Better yesterdays
Laughter some jest
Today bereft
Of the power to change
The drab drab winter day.

So then I thought and laughed
A while
At the drabness so misty grey
On that dreary winter day
And quietly youth returned
Brazen and renewed.

Synaesthesia?

Was it blood
Or were there tears
Or was it rain
Tumbling down
Turning my face
Into a frown
Pushing me
Further
Into the ground –
All I heard
Was silent rain
The taste of blood
Sweet as tears
Bitter and bold.

Laura Hargrove Schneilin

Release

Death came as no surprise
As I wandered by and by
It just shook me from the skies
And left me hanging from on high.

Skeletons

An image lost
Came tumbling back
I washed it out
And lost myself
In memories so cold
I froze to the bone
Images returned
I cleansed my bones
The marrow still drenched
In impossible returns.

Laura Hargrove Schneilin

Manège enchanté

Time wasted
In indolence
In shame
Time found
In happiness
In games
Time lost
In innocence
In despair.

Disgrace

Slow and unbecoming
Images of grief
Came fleeting all around
Grey grim
Sunshine slowly waning
Light falling again
Leaves me unseemly unbelieving.

Blind

I was unable to foresee
Or to predict
Your swinging thoughts
So I rise to nothing
Dash all hope
Resist all change
Incapable of removing
Thoughts of you
Swinging
Right through me
And through you
I know.
Repeat, recall,
Try to forget.

Keep Dreaming

I seek oblivion
From every day
And every feeling
That ever took hold of me.

I seek forgetfulness
From every joy
From every pain
That ever sat beside me.

I may yet seek
For things beyond me.
And then give up,
Silence blessing me.

Laura Hargrove Schneilin

Nox

Motel off the highway
I feel shiftless but can't be
The walls could be shouting
I couldn't hear them
I no longer hear you.

So much here, so clear
The picture, the sight,
Of stairways crunching
Of sheets still squeaking
Newly washed
Still damp for me.

It's your voice I can't hear.
O then, then...
You were so nervous my dear,
You should have been in love.

As

So god fell
And left me.
Standing but reeling
My hands
Can't reach
My throat.

Reeling in darkness
Which never lifts
I wish you
Could reach
My throat.

Laura Hargrove Schneilin

Shards

A tiny ball of hope – so tiny and so frail
–
Resides in every soul in every stone in
Every tree. Release comes O so slowly
Yet springtime never fails.

Carrousel

Twinkle twinkle in my mind
There never was a spark like yours.
Shine on silver grey diamond
I couldn't disbelieve.

Shine on twinkle blue grey star,
You gave it all and then
You took it back.
I keep turning.

Shine on shine on in my mind,
You twinkle like sweet breath,
Twinkle on I might forget
The passing zephyr in my head.

Laura Hargrove Schneilin

II. Love in, Love out

Perfect Fit

You fit me
Like a fist
When I was
Your glove.
Smooth and slippery
You and I,
Which was which?
The fit so tight,
The fist so Lithe,
I fit you
Like a glove
The fit so close
To love.

Repete

Don't die

Don't lie

Don't cry

Take me up

And promise

Conquering

Seeing through

Darkness

The darkness

That made us

Lie

And cry

Laura Hargrove Schneilin

And die

And seem so young.

We should forget

The youth

Silliness

Keep the vibrancy

Lose the vacancy.

So take me in your arms

And die

For a while

And lie

For a while

And cry

Just for me.

Andrzej

Waking up in your arms

Long, lean, unbending

I watch silently as you

Sleep

Silently, undisturbed,
unmoved,

Blond and dirty,

Then I

Watch your sleep

Beer filled but quiet

And think of dreaming

Of the love you give

And take,

Take and give,

Soothed a while I collapse

Laura Hargrove Schneilin

In your sleepy hands.

Red Light

So violent

So vile

Unable

To find

Meaning

In style

He searches

For comfort

In liquid

Divine.

Laura Hargrove Schneilin

Destined part

Only once in your life

Were you meant for me

Once beside me

And inside me

Then alighting

With the dull dim day.

Only once in your life

Was I a flower for you

All too fragrant

And too blatant

To become a trap for you.

So now we kiss and go.

December

I danced with your lips

As if they were mine:

I led and you followed,

First biting then

Smoothing

And then you

Took over.

The dance became yours

And I overwhelmed

Could only succumb

To the lips of a child

I once had called

Mine.

Laura Hargrove Schneilin

Wissen

Not knowing

Who you really are

Is perhaps worse

Than remembering

That night

When you gave

Not knowing

What I took.

Knowing

The end

Is perhaps better

BROKEN SYNTAX

Than perceiving

That moment

Of recovery:

You gave

You took

And left.

Laura Hargrove Schneilin

One Month

It hasn't been a month

The stinging is turning

To dull melancholy.

It's been three weeks.

The bite is but a vague

Remembrance

Of an embrace

Too short of love

Too full of the lust

We desired.

I'd probably forget

If we'd been but playing

With rules.

BROKEN SYNTAX

I remember

Because of your silence

Which said more than

Words.

So I was mistaken

For once and for all.

Laura Hargrove Schneilin

Springtime

Sunshine and bitterness

Carve out the day.

Longing and brittleness

Opened the month of May.

Forlorn or dismayed

I groped through the blankness

How I wish you had stayed –

With you gone I'm a mess.

Epithalamion

I fell a long time

Through the deep deep anger

Of your knocks.

It took the form

Of an ancient abyss

Adorned with knives

White hot none

Too sharp.

And yet I

Held on

To the blades

For fear of falling

To the bottom

Of the ancient abyss.

I still fell and

Broke myself

On the fear and rot

Of your anger.

I couldn't stop

The blood

Running, dripping

Down my eyes

And my cheeks.

The blood was warm

BROKEN SYNTAX

And tranquil

And I hung on.

Laura Hargrove Schneilin

Mage

If I could

Lift you

Out of my thoughts

Then days

Would glide off me

Like days

Should.

But now

I'm drowning

Confounded.

I can't think

Of anything

Beyond

BROKEN SYNTAX

Your pain.

You hurt me yet

I love you:

Quit hurting

That I may live.

Blood

A sugary, useless

Drumbeating heart

Kept mine in thrall

And cleft it apart.

Two wolf-like, bleeding

Starving steel eyes

Tearing me limb to soul

Are departed now gone.

Summertime

This time was love

No in no out

Calm collected

Doubtless.

Eyes wide open

Watching summertime

And summertime.

No doubt

But talking to the wind

Quiet at last

No thoughts but you.

Laura Hargrove Schneilin

Demise

When you left

I died.

But you never left:

You just killed me.

I remember

Reeling, careening,

My stomach acid-filled,

The ups, the downs,

Of being swallowed

Alive

By a dry cold furnace.

Fracture

If I think of you,

Something will be lost

In me

Forever.

The decay

The drab

The unholy alliance

Of sadness and strength

Still shatter me.

Laura Hargrove Schneilin

You Still

You gave me trouble

And love

And the love was troubled

And hate

And the hate was loving

And now we have grief

And long long silences

Full of words unspeakable

But thought and then

Audible but too late.

You gave me love

And all the hardship

The best of both

I cannot choose

BROKEN SYNTAX

Between regret

And forgiveness.

Laura Hargrove Schneilin

S.P.

Out of the mind

And back into darkness

Propelled again

You slowly fall

Out of the grim surroundings

Into some new light

That has no sense

Either

And no certainty yet.

Still back to the mind

To wait and to see

To know and believe

Something for me.

BROKEN SYNTAX